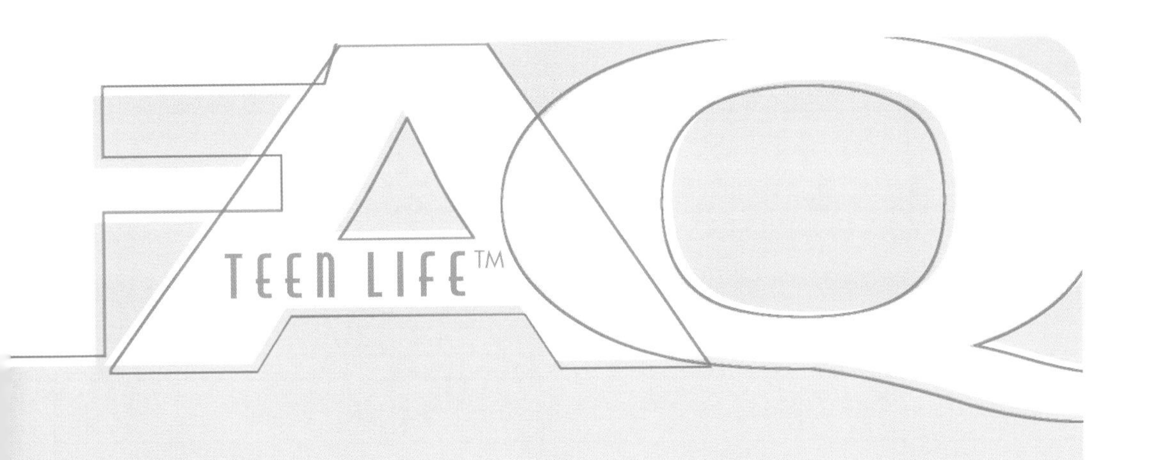

FREQUENTLY ASKED QUESTIONS ABOUT

Sleep and Sleep Deprivation

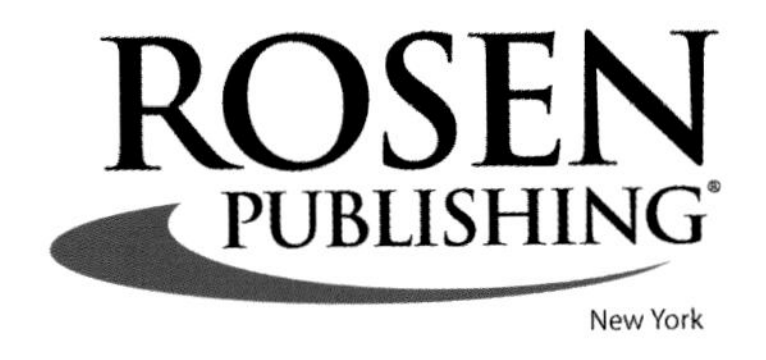

To my mom

Published in 2010 by The Rosen Publishing Group, Inc.
29 East 21st Street, New York, NY 10010

First Edition

Library of Congress Cataloging-in-Publication Data

Peterson, Judy Monroe.
Frequently asked questions about sleep and sleep deprivation / Judy Monroe Peterson.—1st ed.
p. cm.—(FAQ: teen life)
Includes index.
ISBN 978-1-4358-3512-2 (library binding)
1. Sleep. 2. Sleep deprivation. I. Title.
RA786.P48 2010
616.8'498—dc22

2009015481

Manufactured in Malaysia

CPSIA Compliance Information: Batch #TWW10YA: For Further Information contact Rosen Publishing, New York, New York at 1-800-237-9932

Contents

pt one

WHY IS SLEEP IMPORTANT?

Sleep is a state during which most animals and all people, including you, are unaware of their surroundings. It is a natural and biological need, just like the need for food and water. Most people will spend about one-third of their lives sleeping. While sleeping, your eyes are closed, your muscles are relaxed, and your breathing is regular. You typically sleep lying down.

Animals in hibernation are not sleeping. Hibernation is a state of lower metabolism that some animals enter during the winter. The animals cannot awaken while in this state. A sleeping animal or person must be able to wake up. Do you need the loud buzz of an alarm clock to awaken, or can you easily wake up without an alarm clock?

No one can go for too many days and nights without sleep. Like eating right and exercising, getting enough

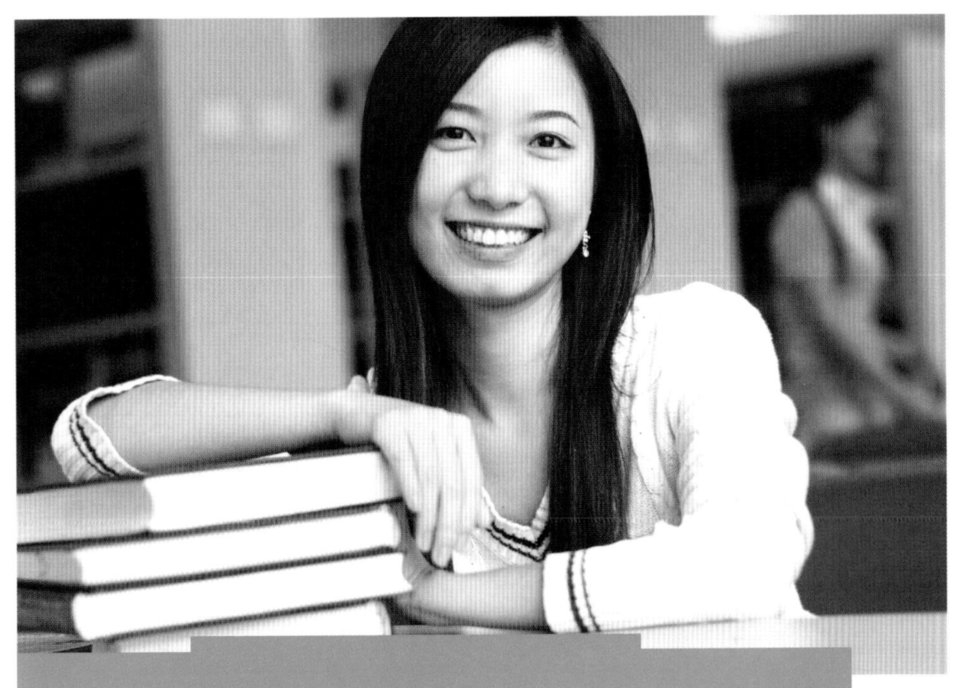

Want to look your best? One thing you can do is to get enough restful sleep every night. Try to keep regular sleep and wake times.

sleep is required for growth, regaining strength, and thinking clearly. Sleep helps you feel better. It affects every aspect of life, including learning, memory, mood, and behavior. A healthy lifestyle requires adequate and restful sleep.

Without a good night's sleep, you will probably feel tired and grumpy. You may have difficulty taking tests or remembering information. It may seem harder than usual to work on school assignments. Tired teens might fall asleep during classes or while driving. Not enough or poor-quality sleep can lead to problems in many aspects of life.

Importance of Sleep

During the day, you use a lot of energy in school, doing schoolwork, and interacting with friends and family. You might play sports, be in clubs or on teams, and have hobbies. You might also have a part-time job. At the end of the day, you usually feel tired and will need to sleep. However, your body and brain are not completely at rest. Sleep is a very active process.

While sleeping, the brain reviews events that happened during the day, processes memories, and makes some of the recent memories more permanent. Sleep helps you learn, reason, and maintain control over your emotions or feelings. Your brain sometimes works out answers to concerns that were troubling you during the day. The answers might surface upon awakening. Have you heard people say they are going to sleep on some problem or decision? Sleeping on an issue may be helpful because the brain processes information and puts different connections together that lead to new insights.

The pituitary gland produces human growth hormone, which is released during sleep. About the size of a pea, the pituitary gland lies under the brain near the center of the skull. A biochemical called growth hormone is produced by the pituitary gland to regulate the growth of children and teens and to help control the way that food is used (metabolism) in people of all ages. It stimulates the growth and replacement of body cells and tissues, and it controls many organs and body functions. In addition, the hormone helps the body to repair itself by healing bruises and wounds.

While you sleep, your immune system is enhanced. The immune system helps your body fight infection caused by bacteria or viruses. Getting plenty of sleep can help you recover from an illness. When you don't get enough sleep, your immune system is temporarily changed. For example, the number of lymphocytes decreases. Lymphocytes are white blood cells that help fight off certain infections.

Sleep lowers stress and helps you feel positive instead of depressed or anxious. Being awake requires energy. During sleep, energy is conserved (saved). Your metabolism slows, and your body temperature falls. You still use some energy during sleep, but less than when you are awake and active.

A Good Night's Sleep

Getting a good night's sleep means that you feel rested, refreshed, and alert. You have energy for the coming day. You awake on time and don't hit the snooze button repeatedly. Restful sleep provides many benefits. Teens who get enough sleep typically perform better than those who do not. They usually don't procrastinate (put off doing things) because they are too tired.

Getting enough sleep is associated with improved memory and creativity. You are better able to deal with the ups and downs of life and solving everyday problems. For example, if you have test anxiety, you might decide to ask the school counselor for help in learning test-taking techniques. Instead of juggling school, work, and odd jobs to pay for gas for a car, you can look into other ways to get places. You might decide that bicycling, walking, taking the bus, or carpooling are good alternatives. You can think of better solutions to problems when you're rested.

Minor health problems may disappear with good sleep. Teens who are constantly tired might experience frequent headaches or stomach discomfort. They also get sick with colds or the flu more often. Another benefit is that teens may find that maintaining a healthy weight is easier when they get enough sleep.

Stages of Sleep

Sleep is an orderly process. Your body goes through sleep cycles. Teens typically go through four or five full cycles during the night. Each cycle lasts about sixty to ninety minutes and goes through five stages of sleep.

Each sleep cycle has two states: rapid eye movement (REM) and non-REM. REM is the dream state, and non-REM is quiet sleep. The sleep cycle goes from light non-REM sleep, to deep non-REM sleep, and then to REM sleep. The cycle occurs about every ninety minutes during the night. Teens spend most of the night in non-REM sleep. During this state, the body repairs and energizes itself. Brain waves become slower, reaching their slowest and deepest level during Stage IV.

Non-REM Sleep

Non-REM sleep is made up of four stages. Stage I, called light sleep, lasts about five minutes. Stage II, or the onset of sleep, lasts thirty to forty minutes. During Stage I and Stage II, your

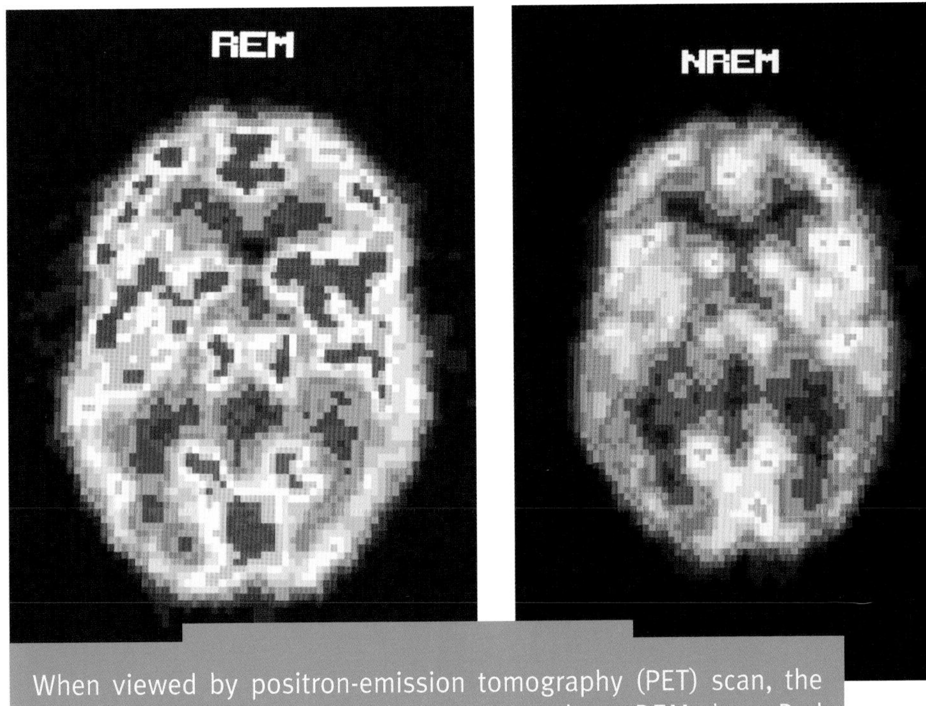

When viewed by positron-emission tomography (PET) scan, the human brain looks different during REM and non-REM sleep. Red shows the active areas of the brain during REM sleep. Inactive areas are blue.

brain waves slow, and your heart rate and body temperature drop. People can be easily woken during these stages.

Stage III and Stage IV are deep-sleep stages. Brain waves become slower and larger. Heart rate and breathing slow and become more regular. Teens spend about 20 to 25 percent of their sleep time in deep sleep. During this state, less blood goes to the brain. Growth hormone is released, which stimulates the growth and repair of muscles and wounds. The immune system is also enhanced during this time. It's more difficult to wake people up when they are in Stage IV sleep.

REM Sleep

REM sleep occurs after the non-REM stages. REM sleep is also called the dream state. Teens typically spend more than two hours each night dreaming. During REM sleep, your body barely moves because the muscles that move your body go limp. Your brain is active, and your eyes dart back and forth or up and down during dreams. Your heart rate, breathing rate, blood pressure, and brain waves rise and fall with the action in your dreams. REM sleep occurs about every ninety minutes and lasts five to thirty minutes. You have more (longer) REM sleep in the later part of the night.

Sometimes, nightmares happen during REM sleep. These frightening dreams may awaken you. If awoken from REM sleep, you are more likely to remember your nightmare or dream.

Researchers are not sure why people dream and have nightmares. Some think that dreams are how the brain tries to find meaning from the various signals it receives during REM sleep. Dreaming sleep is involved in restoring the brain's ability to handle tasks like concentration, learning, and memory. Most people only remember a small portion of their dreams. Some don't remember any of their dreams.

Circadian Rhythm

In addition to sleep cycles, your circadian rhythm plays a key part in the timing of sleep. The body has a circadian, or approximately twenty-four-hour, cycle of sleep and wakefulness. You

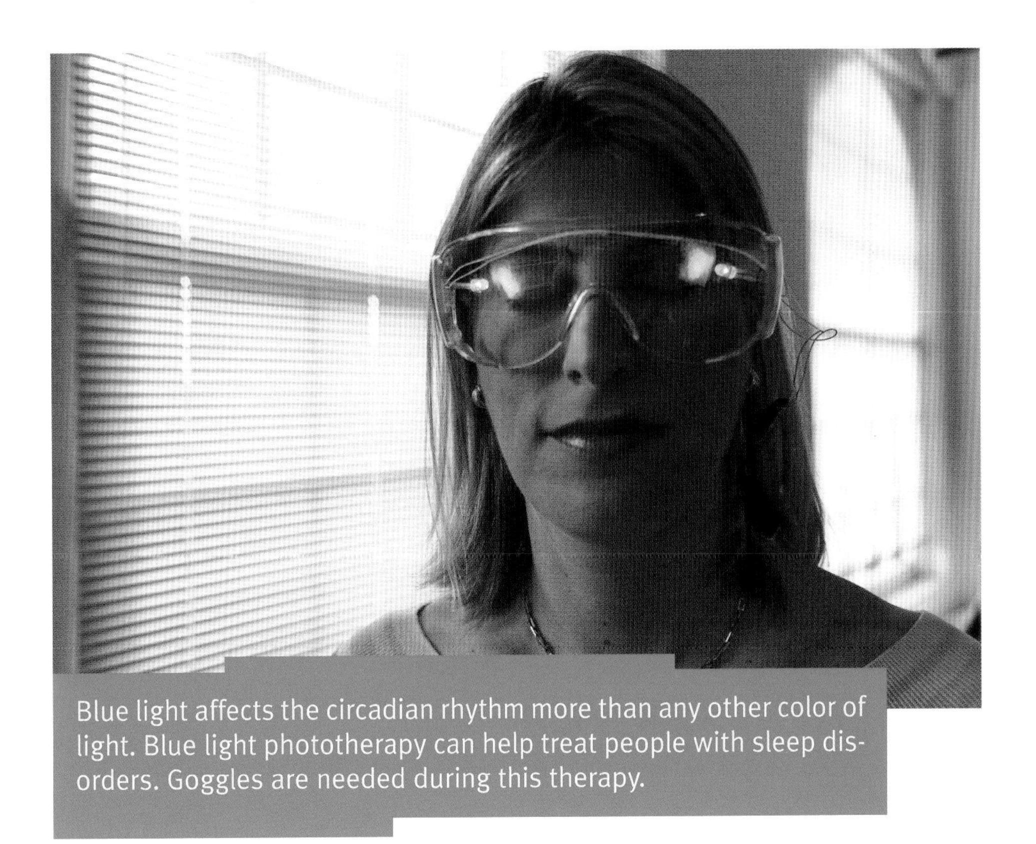

Blue light affects the circadian rhythm more than any other color of light. Blue light phototherapy can help treat people with sleep disorders. Goggles are needed during this therapy.

are awake and active during the day when there is sunlight. You sleep at night when the sun has set and there is darkness.

The circadian rhythm is regulated by a clock inside your body. Every person has a built-in, or biological, clock that regulates sleeping and waking. This biological clock is found in the suprachiasmatic nucleus (SCN), which is a small group of cells in the center of the brain. When it is nighttime and dark, no light enters the eyes. The SCN then sends messages to the pineal gland to produce the hormone melatonin. When melatonin flows into the brain, you get sleepy. When light shines in your eyes during the day, the SCN sends signals to the pineal gland to stop producing melatonin, and you feel more alert.

Your circadian rhythm is also controlled by body temperature. Your body temperature has a twenty-four-hour cycle. It rises during the day, dips in the late afternoon, and then climbs again. By nighttime, your body temperature begins to drop again. It's lowest at about four o'clock in the morning. After that, your body starts getting ready to wake up, so your body temperature begins increasing.

The biological clock of some people does not follow the typical circadian cycle. Instead, they feel most awake in the late afternoon, evening, or at night. They cannot fall asleep until two or three o'clock in the morning. If they must get up early in the morning, they feel tired and have low energy. People, though, might feel tired when they wake up because they have another sleep problem or a sleep disorder.

pt two

ARE YOU GETTING ENOUGH SLEEP?

According to the National Sleep Foundation, most teens require about nine hours or more of sleep each night. Some may need only eight-and-a-half hours, while others may need up to ten hours. However, many teens average about six-and-a-half hours, and some try to get by on six hours or less.

Compared to adults, teens require more sleep because they are developing rapidly. Sleep is especially important during growth spurts of two or more inches (five or more centimeters) a year. If you don't get enough sleep, you could experience a variety of problems.

Reasons for Not Getting Enough Sleep

Many teens don't get enough sleep because they don't often understand the importance of sleep for good mental

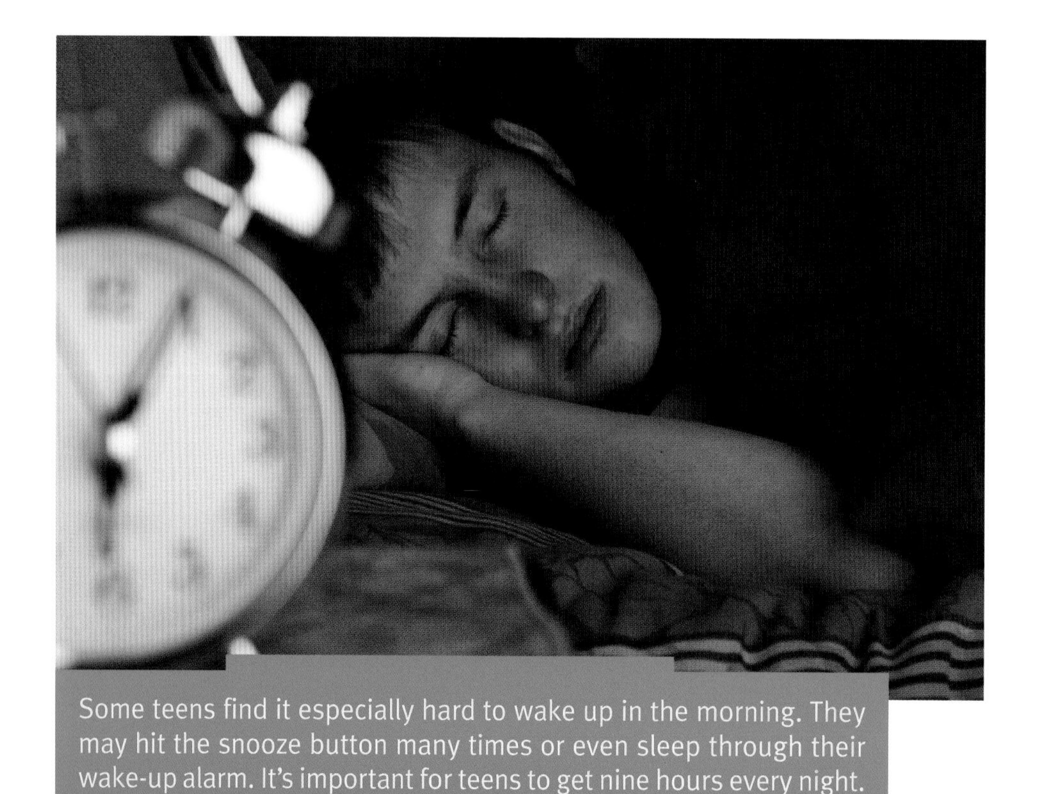

Some teens find it especially hard to wake up in the morning. They may hit the snooze button many times or even sleep through their wake-up alarm. It's important for teens to get nine hours every night.

and physical health. Quite a number of teens are overscheduled and try to cram in too many activities. They go to school, do schoolwork, play sports, work part-time jobs, and are members of clubs and teams. They take time for phone calls, instant messaging, and the Internet. Teens spend time with friends and family, helping at home, and doing other activities like band, hobbies, listening to music, or watching television. If you typically squeeze in as many activities every day as possible, you might not be getting enough sleep.

Early-start school can cause sleep problems for some teens. Most high schools start between 7:00 and 8:00 AM. To be on time, teens need to wake between 5:30 and 6:30 AM. If they were up until midnight or later the night before, they will not get enough sleep.

Teens might change their sleeping patterns during the week, but this can cause sleep problems. For example, on school nights, you might stay up late and then get up early for school. On Friday and Saturday nights, you might stay awake even later to be with friends. Then you sleep in late on Saturday and Sunday, or you may need to get up in the morning for religious or family events. Having different sleep patterns might seem like a good idea. However, you function best if you follow your biological clock. Constantly changing sleep patterns throws off the circadian rhythm of your body.

Other factors can contribute to not getting enough sleep. Although illegal, some teens drink alcohol. Alcohol interferes with REM and non-REM cycles, resulting in teens not getting enough REM and deep sleep. Drugs, including caffeine and the nicotine in tobacco products, lessen the amount of REM sleep for users. Many illegal drugs, such as marijuana and cocaine, can also cause serious sleep problems. It's common for people to get very excited about an event and then have difficulty falling asleep the night before. Other strong emotions, such as anxiety, anger, or depression, can keep people from falling or staying asleep. Then they wake up feeling groggy and tired.

Sleep Deprivation and Sleep Debt

You are sleep deprived if you feel drowsy or tired during the day. Even if a teacher or a movie in class is boring, you should not nod off or fall asleep at your desk. Other signs of sleep deprivation include difficulty getting up for school and struggling to stay awake while doing schoolwork or other activities during the day or evening.

Some people are so sleep deprived that they have microsleeps. These moments of sleep occur when they are awake and their eyes are open. Usually, people have no memory of experiencing microsleeps.

If you don't get enough sleep, you will accumulate a sleep debt. For example, if you lose one hour of sleep for five nights in a row, your sleep debt builds to five hours. You might try to make up your debt by sleeping most of Saturday morning. However, sleeping extra hours on the weekend may not completely reverse the effects of sleep deprivation during the week. To get out and stay out of debt, you need to sleep as much as your body needs every night.

Sleep Deprivation and Performance, Mood, and Health

Sleep deprivation affects every part of daily life, resulting in short-term and long-term consequences. Just one night of inadequate sleep can alter functioning and mood the next day. If sleep deprived, teens have less ability to concentrate, learn, and recall what they have learned. They have more injuries and accidents at school, home, and work. They are less alert and creative, and they have more mood and behavioral problems.

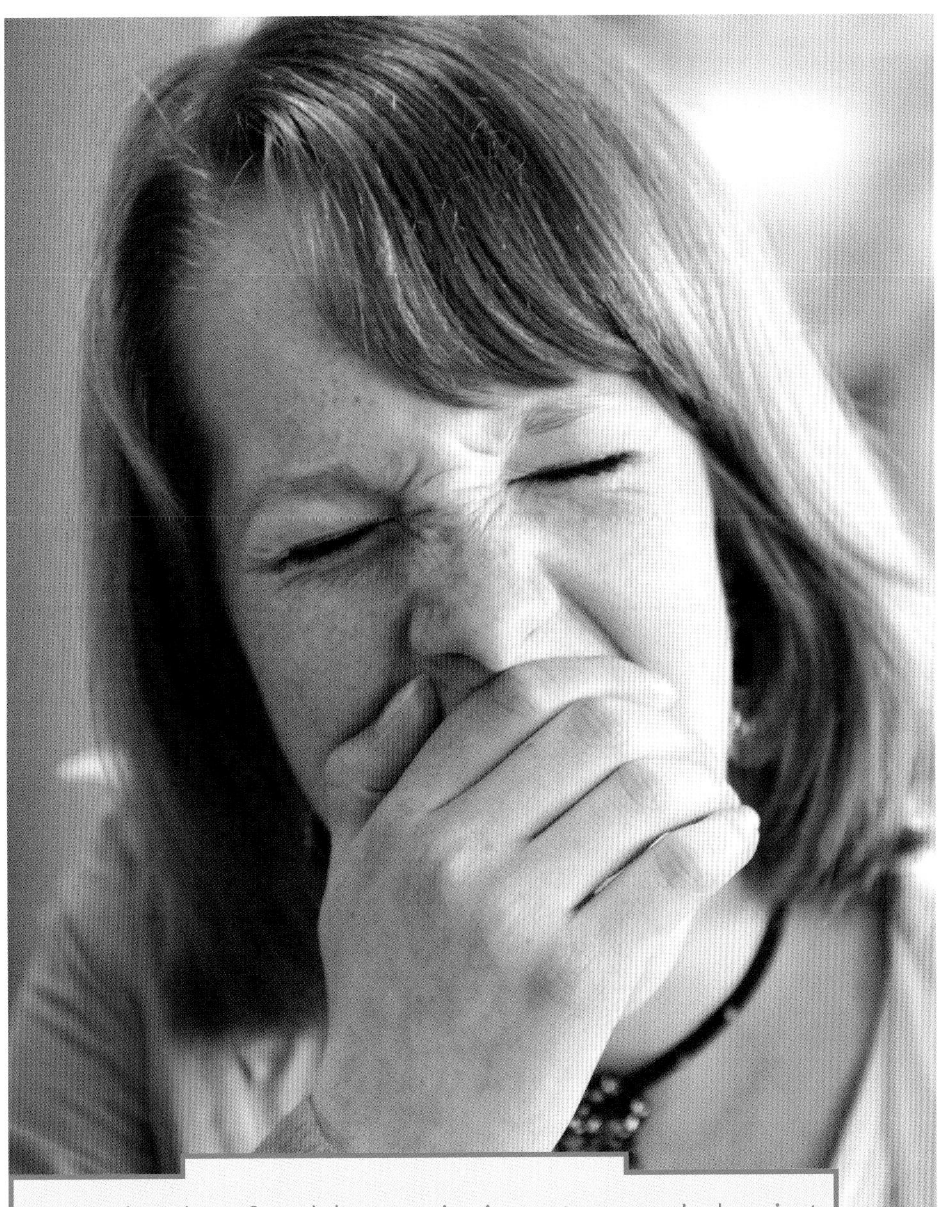

Researchers have found that yawning is most commonly done just before and after sleeping. If sleepy teens yawn during classes, they might be close to falling asleep. Getting good sleep helps teens stay awake during the day.

Lack of sleep affects performance in school, often resulting in lower grades. Tired teens tend to make more spelling and math errors and have more difficulty remembering information. Learning, thinking processes, and memory pathways in the brain slow down. Being tired makes it difficult to focus and pay attention.

Teens who are sleep deprived may feel negative and have poor control over their emotions. They may be irritable, unhappy, angry, and impatient. Some become more aggressive. Others become depressed. Tired teens often have increased problems with peer and adult relationships and handling social activities.

Lack of sleep has an impact on overall health. If you are sleep deprived, you will not look your best. Your eyes will be droopy, and there might be dark circles underneath them. Sleep deprivation can make skin problems like acne or eczema worse. You will get sick more often and have more frequent headaches and aches and pains. According to the National Institutes of Health, the current epidemic of obesity and diabetes may be due, in part, to sleep deprivation. Sleep helps regulate appetite, energy use, and weight. People who are continually tired are more likely to be overweight and eat high-calorie foods. As a result, they have a greater chance of developing diabetes and other chronic health problems.

Sports, Driving, and Sleepy Teens

Sleepy teens have less endurance, strength, and speed. This can affect their performance in activities like sports. Inadequate sleep can lead to slower reaction time, poor decision making and

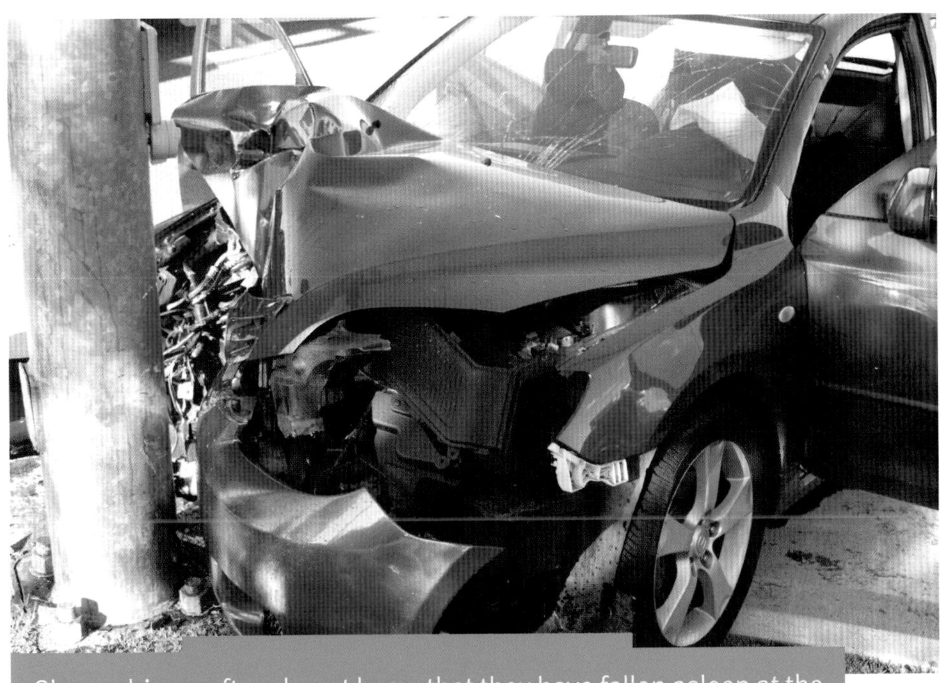

Sleepy drivers often do not know that they have fallen asleep at the wheel. When asleep, drivers lose control of their cars. Accidents can then happen fast.

problem solving, and increased risk taking. For example, although you are tired, you might decide to take a long drive.

Sleepy drivers are at increased risk of causing or being in an accident. They may have trouble keeping their eyes focused on the road, or they may fall asleep at the wheel. People are often unaware that they have briefly slept while driving. The response time of sleepy drivers may be too slow to avoid an unexpected road problem. Traffic accidents can result in injury to people, vehicles, and other property—and it can result in death. According to the National Highway Traffic Safety Administration, a main cause of traffic deaths is driving while tired. It only takes a few seconds to fall asleep and lose control of the car. If you feel sleepy while driving, pull off the road in a safe place and nap fifteen to twenty minutes.

Stimulants and Sleep

Tired teens are more likely to use stimulants than well-rested teens. Stimulants are drugs that make people feel more awake and alert for a short time. They speed up the nervous system and increase the activity of the mind and body. However, regular stimulant use can lead to loss of sleep, resulting in more sleep deprivation.

The caffeine in coffee, tea, cocoa, and some sodas is a stimulant. It's also a common ingredient in pain relievers and cold medicines. Do you drink coffee or sodas with caffeine to wake up in the morning or to stay awake? You may be addicted to caffeine. If you don't get your usual amount of the drug, you may get headaches and feel cross and moody. Nicotine is another stimulant. It causes smokers to sleep lightly and not get restful sleep. Amphetamines, another stimulant, are useful medical drugs. Illegal amphetamines, commonly called "meth" (methamphetamines), are made in home laboratories. Use of amphetamines without a doctor's prescription is dangerous and can cause serious problems, even death.

Getting Too Much Sleep

Sometimes, teens may be getting too much sleep. This could be a sign of a disease like mononucleosis, also called "mono" or "the kissing disease." This disease is caused by the Epstein-Barr virus. The main symptoms are fever, sore throat, headaches, swollen glands in the neck, not feeling hungry, abdominal discomfort, and feeling tired. The symptoms of mononucleosis usually go away on their own after three to four weeks. Teens who have mono need plenty of sleep to get well.

Teens who sleep too much or too little might be feeling tense, bored, or depressed. People who are depressed feel sad, hopeless, and tired. Their depression causes them to lose interest in school, friends, and social activities. They cannot deal well with everyday life. Depression can be a serious medical illness that requires treatment. It can also be a sign of drug abuse, drug addiction, or sleep disorders. An actual sleep disorder might also be a cause of sleeping too much.

Chapter three

WHAT ARE COMMON TEEN SLEEP DISORDERS?

Sleep is automatic and natural for most people. They fall asleep easily, sleep through the night, and wake up in the morning feeling rested and refreshed. For other people, getting a good night's sleep is not easy. For example, you might have difficulty falling asleep, or you might wake up often at night and cannot fall back to sleep quickly. If you wake up tired and lack energy, you may not be getting as much sleep as your body needs. You may have a sleep problem. An occasional night of poor sleep happens to everyone. However, if these problems go on for two weeks or longer, you might have a sleep disorder.

According to the National Institutes of Health, 30 to 40 percent of people in the United States have sleep disorders. Some people report that they developed their sleep

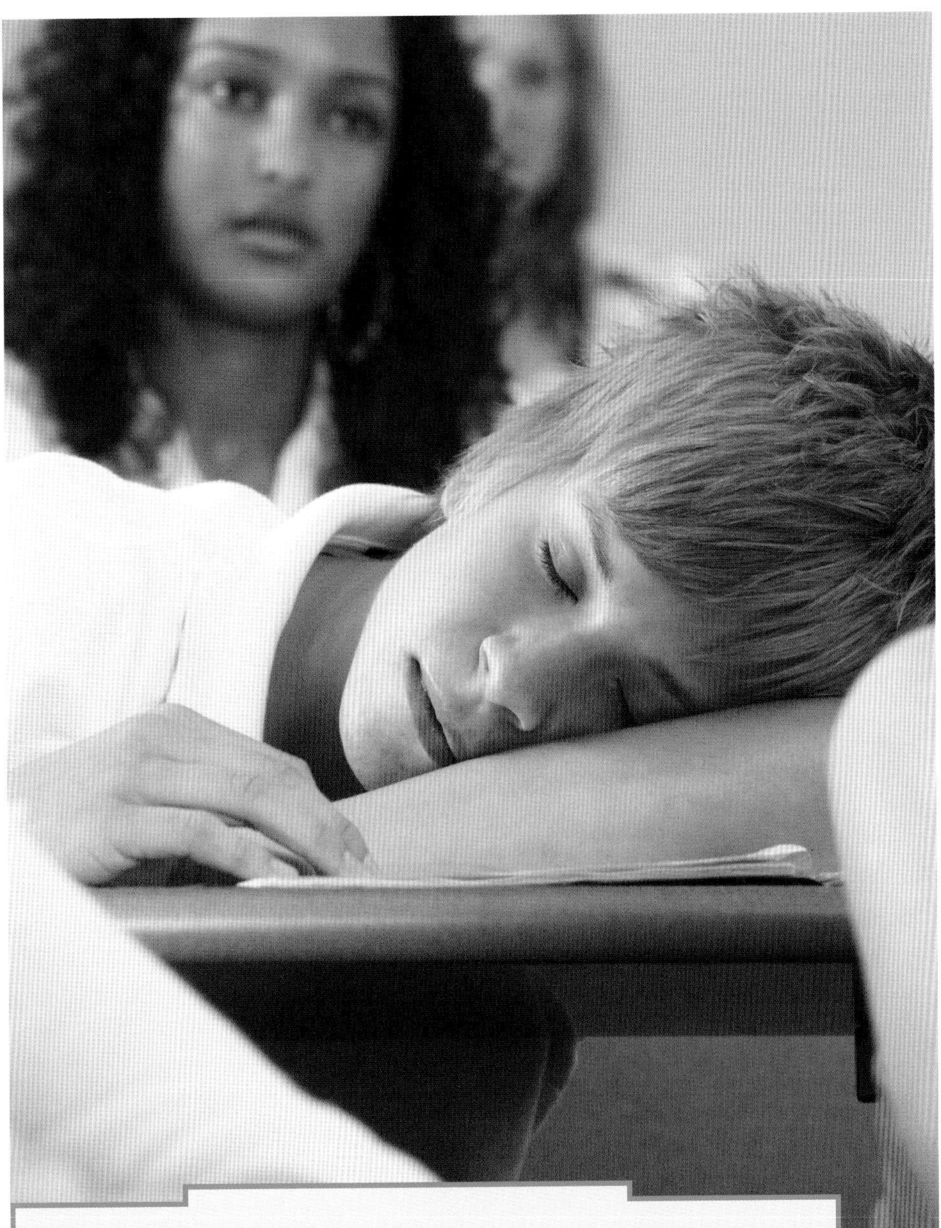

Teens who usually do not get enough sleep or sleep poorly are tired. They may doze off in class. As a result, they may do poorly on tests and get low grades.

problem during their teen years. Doctors have documented more than seventy sleep disorders. The ones that most commonly affect teens are insomnia, sleep apnea, delayed sleep phase syndrome, restless legs syndrome, and narcolepsy. Sometimes, sleepwalking is a problem for teens, too.

Signs of Sleep Disorders

Read over this list of common signs of sleep disorders. If you have any of the following signs for two weeks or longer, see your family doctor:

- Difficulty getting asleep, staying asleep, or waking up too early
- Not feeling rested when awake
- Feeling sleepy or dozing off during the day
- People saying that you snore, gasp, choke, or stop breathing during sleep
- Having creepy, crawly, or tingling feelings in your legs
- Feeling that you cannot move when you first wake up
- Drinking a lot of coffee or sodas with caffeine to stay awake during the day
- Difficulty focusing, concentrating, and remembering new information
- Feeling more tired and irritable as the day goes on

It's important to seek medical attention if you're having any of these feelings or problems, as there are usually good interventions for sleep issues.

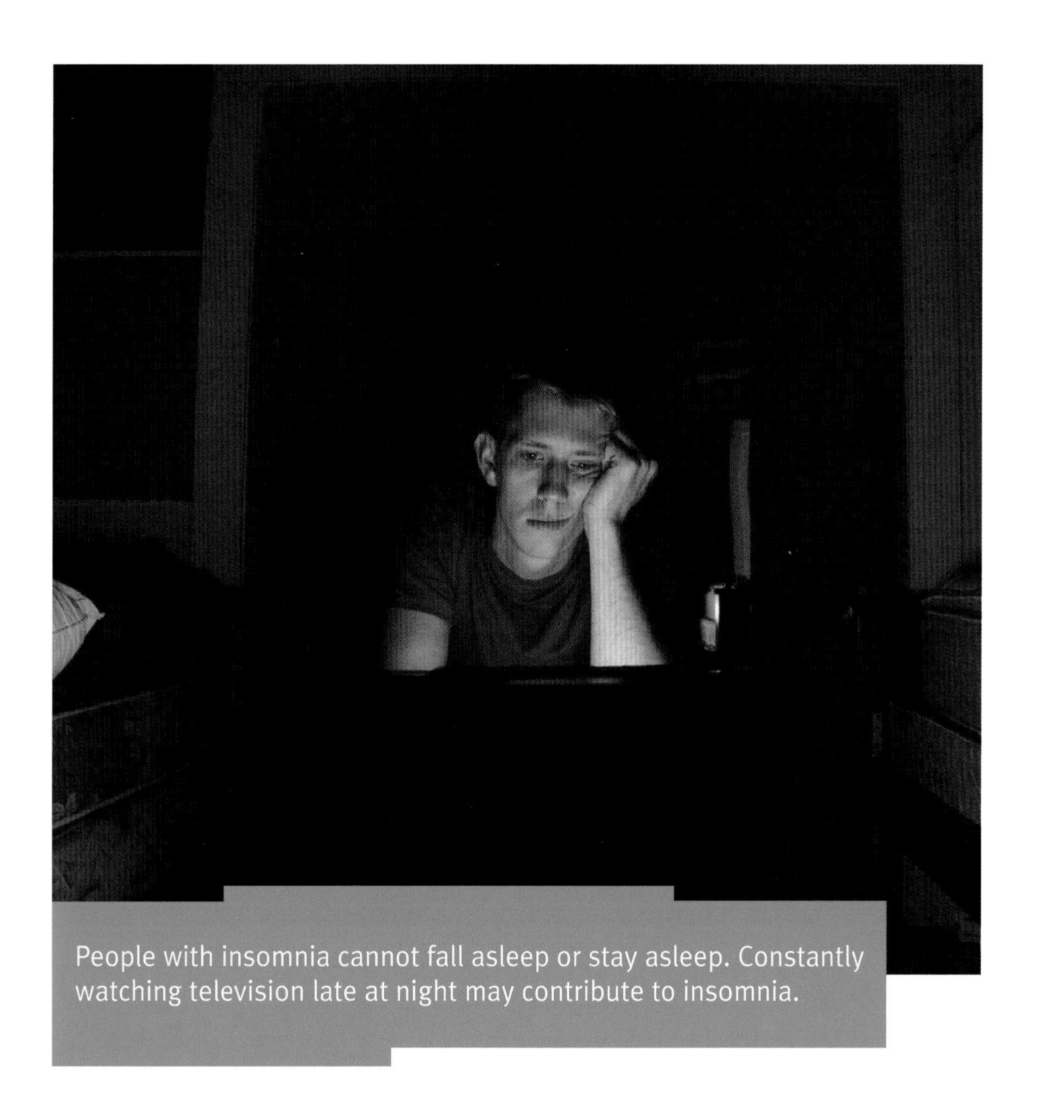

People with insomnia cannot fall asleep or stay asleep. Constantly watching television late at night may contribute to insomnia.

Insomnia

Insomnia is the inability to fall asleep or stay asleep, or not feeling refreshed when you awaken. It's the most common sleep disorder in the United States. According to the National Institutes of Health, about 10 percent of Americans have insomnia. If you have insomnia, you may feel sleepy, tired, listless, and depressed. You may also feel irritable and have difficulty concentrating and focusing. Short-term insomnia can last one night, several nights, or a few weeks. If your insomnia lasts more than a month, it is called chronic insomnia.

The causes of insomnia vary. Sleep can be disrupted because of noisy neighbors or a loud plane flying overhead. Coughing due to a cold during the night can bring on insomnia. Your bedroom might be too hot or cold, or noisy neighbors might make falling asleep difficult. Many teens experience short-term insomnia due to stress, including family problems, worry over school tests, or relationship issues. A traffic accident or another traumatic event can bring on short-term insomnia. You may become so anxious about not sleeping that your anxiety causes your insomnia to last longer.

Chronic insomnia is often caused by depression or anxiety disorders. Sometimes, chronic insomnia is due to a disease, a sleep disorder, or medications. People with arthritis or asthma tend to have more pain or breathing problems at night, which affects sleep. Some prescription and over-the-counter medicines can cause insomnia, including cold medicines, pain relievers, and steroids.

Sleep Apnea

People with sleep apnea have difficulty breathing during sleep because they have shallow breathing or stop breathing for ten to twenty seconds. This can occur twenty to thirty times each hour.

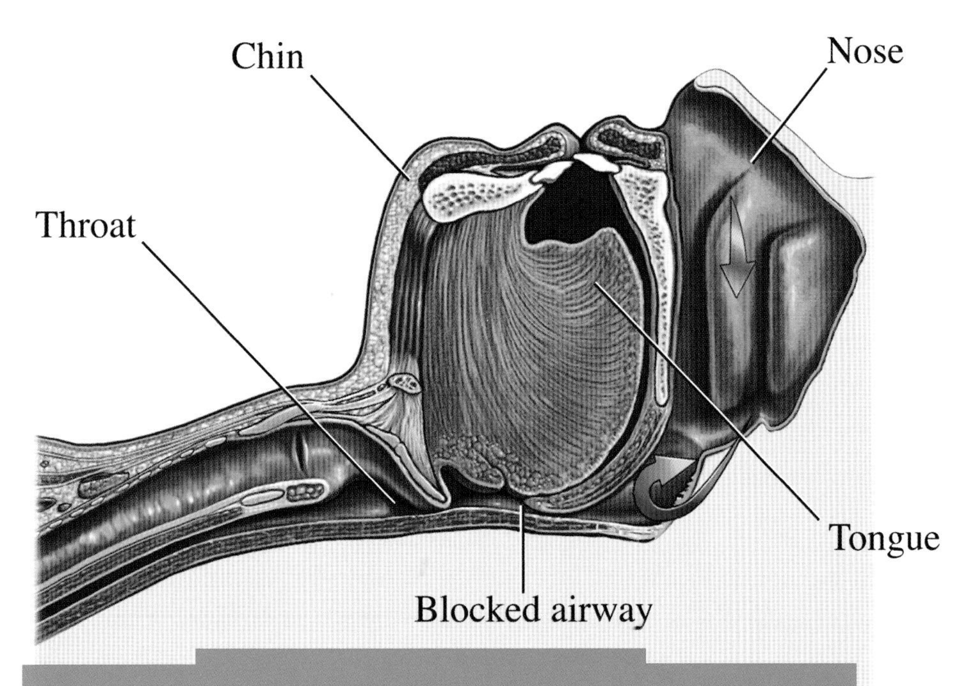

This drawing shows how the upper airway is blocked during obstructive apnea. The tissues of the tongue and throat close off the airway when lying down. Then the lungs do not receive enough oxygen.

When you are not breathing, you wake up to start breathing again. Because you wake up so often during the night, you don't feel refreshed in the morning.

The National Institutes of Health estimate that twelve to eighteen million people in the United States have sleep apnea, and about 3 percent of children and teens have the disorder. There are two general kinds of sleep apnea, central and obstructive. Central apnea is caused by a problem within the brain itself that makes a person "forget" to breathe temporarily. It is much less common than obstructive sleep apnea, which is often caused by tissue that blocks the airways in the throat during sleep. Not enough oxygen comes in through the mouth and nose, and the lungs don't receive enough oxygen. Due to the rise in blood levels of carbon dioxide, you wake up and automatically tighten the muscles around the tissues in your throat. This causes your windpipe to open, and you breathe again. As your breathing begins, you may snort, gasp, or make a choking sound. Loud, frequent snoring is a common sign of sleep apnea.

Sleep apnea interferes with deep sleep. As a result, you may have morning headaches and feel sleepy all day. You may have learning, memory, behavior, and mood problems, such as agitation, aggression, or depression. People tend to have more car accidents. The disorder causes increased amounts of growth hormone and stress hormones to be released, interferes with metabolism, and increases a desire to eat carbohydrates. People with obstructive sleep apnea are often overweight, which leads to extra floppy tissues in the neck and throat that tend to collapse when they fall asleep and results in apnea. People with sleep apnea may have increased blood pressure and heart rates, which increases their risk of developing heart problems and diabetes, and becoming overweight or obese.

Sleepwalking and Sleep Talking

Sleepwalking can be a problem for some teens, but it's uncommon in older teens. It typically occurs within two to three hours after falling asleep, during Stage III or Stage IV deep sleep.

Sleepwalkers may wander around for a few minutes or more, up to thirty minutes. They might sit up in bed and talk or mumble. Sometimes, they slowly walk or shuffle around and open and close doors or drawers. They might get dressed, walk up and down stairs, get and eat food, or use the bathroom.

You can gently guide a sleepwalker back to bed. Don't try to wake sleepwalkers, though. They're difficult to awaken, and they typically have no memory of the event in the morning.

Many people, including teens, talk, laugh, or cry out in their sleep. This typically happens between the non-REM and REM cycles of sleep. Sleep talkers can seem to carry on a conversation. However, they don't realize that they are talking and have no memory of the event when they awake. Doctors don't usually consider sleep talking and sleepwalking as true sleep disorders.

Delayed Sleep Phase Syndrome

Delayed sleep phase syndrome is a disorder of sleep timing. You cannot fall asleep before midnight to 3:00 AM, and you have difficulty waking in the morning. The disorder is rare in adults but common among teens. It can seriously impact everyday life.

Teens with delayed sleep phase syndrome often call themselves "night owls" and can think and learn best in the evening and night. If they try to go to sleep before midnight, they cannot. However, they easily fall asleep at their usual time and will feel rested if they sleep until late morning.

When they get up early for school, teens with this disorder stay sleepy all day. They may take naps or fall asleep in

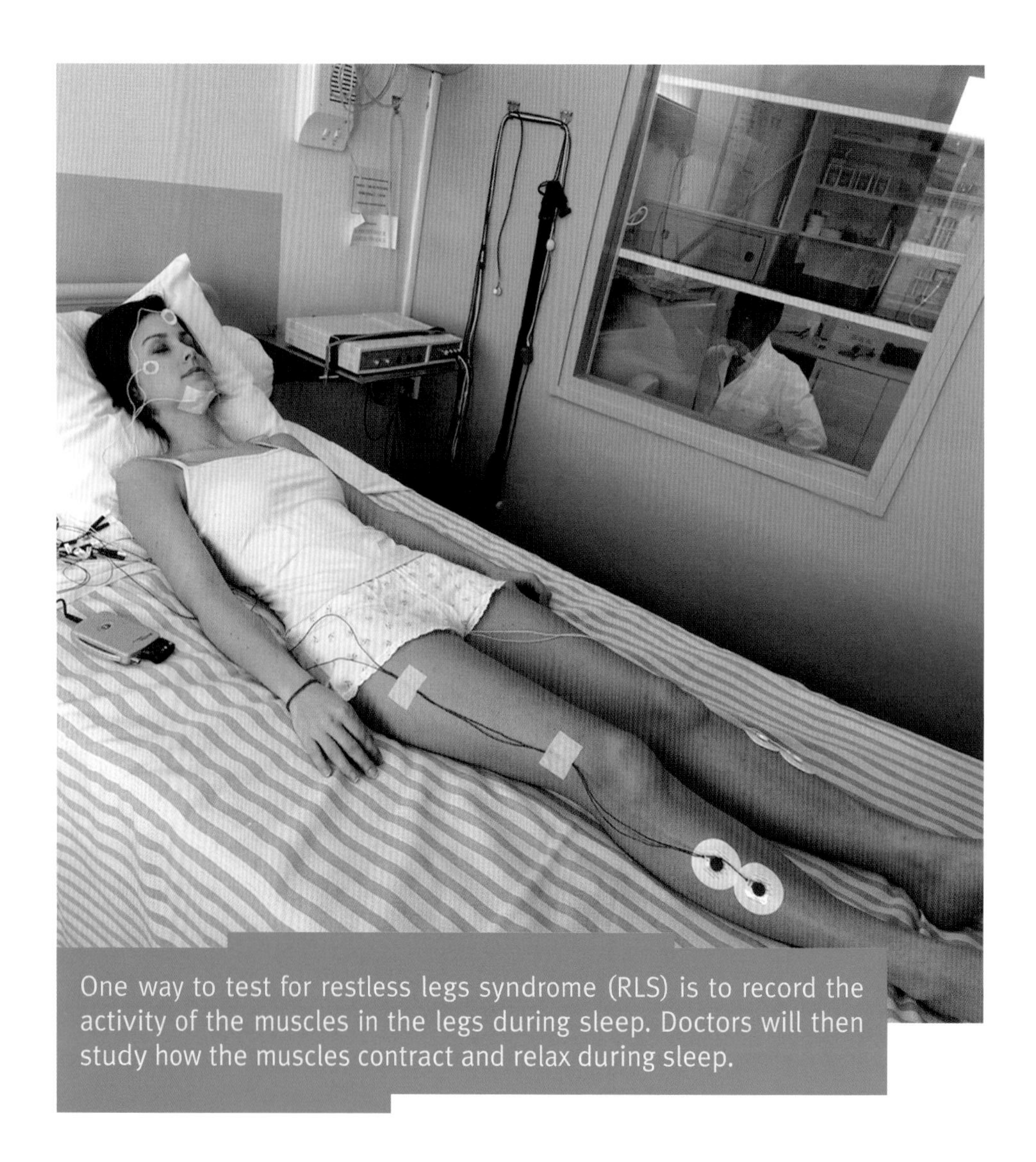

One way to test for restless legs syndrome (RLS) is to record the activity of the muscles in the legs during sleep. Doctors will then study how the muscles contract and relax during sleep.

school, and miss out on social activities or spending time with friends and family. Some experience depression, become moody, and have behavioral problems. Teens usually outgrow this disorder.

Restless Legs Syndrome

Restless legs syndrome (RLS) causes tingling, creepy, gnawing, crawly, tugging, or pulling feelings in the legs and sometimes in the arms. The uncomfortable feelings usually occur in the evening and at bedtime, or when sitting for a long time, such as when working at a desk, watching a movie, or on long rides. People stretch, move, or massage their legs to get rid of the uncomfortable feelings. Because RLS starts or becomes worse when resting or lying down, people may have difficulty falling and staying asleep. RLS is typically worse at the beginning of the night and improves as the night goes on.

Many people who have RLS also have limb movements during sleep that occur every five to ninety seconds. This is called periodic limb movement disorder (PLMD). The jerking legs during sleep often awaken people and reduce their sleep time.

According to the Restless Legs Syndrome Foundation, this disorder affects more than ten million adults and about 1.5 million children and teens in the United States. RLS and PLMD typically begin during childhood or the teen years. RLS is often inherited and is a lifelong condition. Currently, some experimental medicines are being tried for people with severe RLS.

Narcolepsy

Narcolepsy is caused by the inability of the brain to regulate sleep-wake cycles. During the day, people with this disorder feel extremely sleepy and suddenly fall asleep for a few seconds to several minutes or more. "Sleep attacks" can occur at any time and any place without warning. The attacks can cause difficulty in school, with relationships, and at work.

Other symptoms of narcolepsy are cataplexy (sudden muscle weakness) and hallucinations or vivid dreams while going in and out of sleep. Another frightening symptom is the inability to move when you first awake. Most people with narcolepsy wake up many times during the night, although they often can sleep seven or eight hours at night. Narcolepsy is a rare disorder. It typically appears during the teen years and remains for life.

Feeling tired occasionally is normal. However, you may have a medical problem if you are often sleepy during the day and lack energy. You should seek professional help for possible sleep problems or disorders.

Myths and Facts

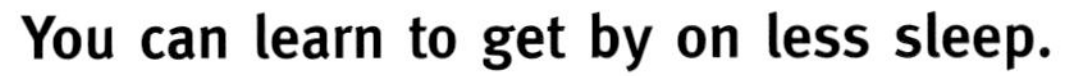

Myth **You can learn to get by on less sleep.**

Fact: You cannot train your body to get by on less sleep than it needs. You may be able to function on less sleep, but you will feel tired and get less done.

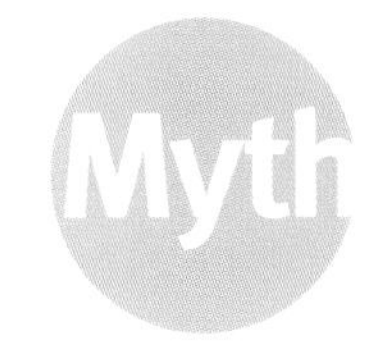

You can get too much sleep.

Fact: Your body needs a certain amount of sleep every night. You cannot get more than that amount because of your circadian rhythm and sleep-wake hormones. If you sleep more than usual, it is because your body needs the extra sleep.

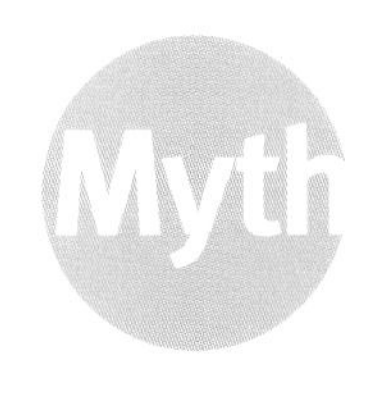

Herbal supplements are a great way to treat insomnia.

Fact: Little scientific evidence exists that herbal supplements can help people with sleep problems. In addition, herbal supplements might interact with medications. Tell your doctor if you are using herbal supplements. In some cases, your doctor may prescribe melatonin for circadian rhythm disturbances, but this medicine should only be taken under his or her direction.

Chapter four

HOW CAN A SLEEP DOCTOR HELP?

If you typically feel sleepy during most days, toss and turn all night, or think you have a sleep disorder, see your family doctor. Your doctor may recommend treatment or refer you to a sleep specialist who can determine if you have a sleep disorder. Sleep doctors use various tools, including an overnight stay at a sleep center, to arrive at a diagnosis and treatment plan.

Family Doctors

See your family doctor if you are sleeping poorly or feel overly tired. At your appointment, talk about your sleep problems. Your doctor will likely take your health history, conduct a physical exam, and request lab tests. Based on the results, your doctor may help you with your sleep problem. For example, you might be sleeping poorly after a traffic accident or a death in the family.

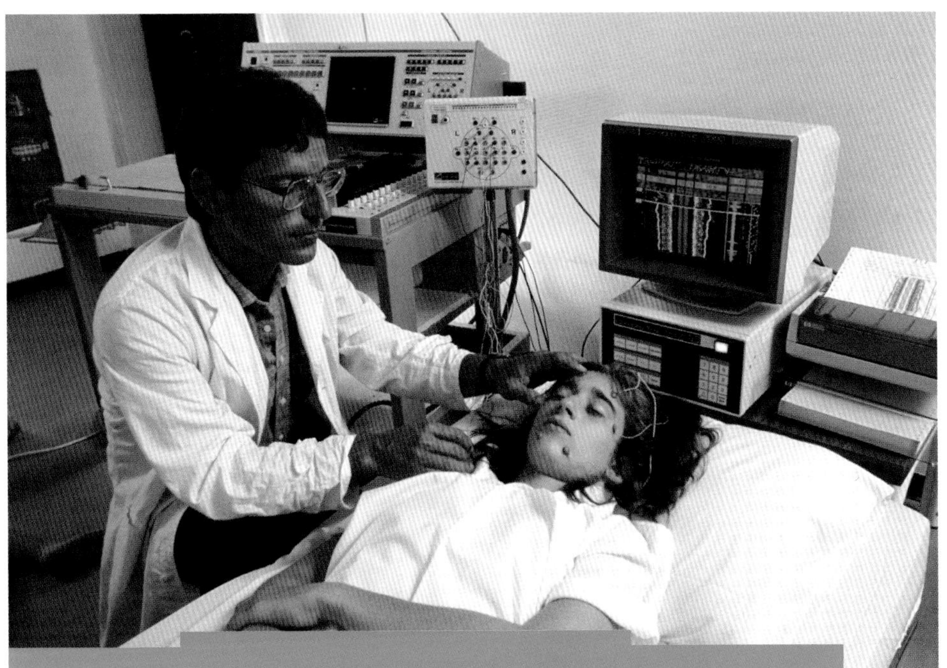

A technician is preparing this teen for a sleep study. He pasted small sensors to the teen's scalp, face, chest, and legs. Now he is attaching thin wires to the sensors.

When you explain your sleep problem to your doctor, you may be prescribed a medicine, such as an antihistamine, for short-term use. Antihistamines often make people sleepy and last through the night.

If you have signs of depression, anxiety, physical abuse, or other issues, your doctor might refer you to a psychologist or psychiatrist for treatment. Your doctor may also run some blood tests to look at your hemoglobin level or thyroid function. Your laboratory tests might show that you have a disease or condition like anemia. The anemia could be caused by a deficiency in iron. If you have anemia, you may feel tired, weak, and dizzy, and have headaches. Treatment depends on the cause of your anemia. You might need iron supplements, for example.

If your doctor suspects that your sleep problems have a medical cause, you will be referred to a sleep specialist. You can also ask your family doctor for a referral to see a sleep specialist. Usually, sleep doctors first train in neurology (study of the nervous system) or pulmonology (study of the respiratory system), then receive extra training to become a sleep specialist. Many work at sleep centers and labs. According to the American Association of Sleep Medicine, more than 1,500 accredited sleep centers are located throughout the United States.

What Sleep Doctors Do

Before you see a sleep specialist, you will receive a list of questions about your sleep history. Complete the questionnaire and bring it to your appointment.

At your appointment, the sleep doctor will ask about your sleep problems and sleep habits. The doctor might ask you to keep a sleep diary for a week or longer. You will use the diary to write daily bedtimes and wake-up times, what medicines you took and when, when you drank beverages with caffeine, and when and how long you napped and exercised. You will also need to report any alcohol or street drug use.

During your next appointment, the sleep specialist will review your diary. The doctor will also ask you about recent stressful issues, medical and family history, allergies, medications, and health habits. In addition, you will answer questions about the likelihood that you randomly fall asleep at different times and places. To get more information, the sleep doctor might have you take a sleep test at a sleep center or lab.

At the Sleep Center

Depending on the tests that your doctor orders, you will be at the sleep center about twelve to eighteen hours. Many of your body functions and movements will be recorded for hours during the test. Sleep tests are painless.

On the day of your sleep study, avoid caffeine and don't nap. You can shower and wash your hair, but don't put anything else in your hair or wear makeup. Pack an overnight bag with your nightclothes, pillow, toothbrush, and clothes for the next day. Bring your regular medications, if you use any.

Sleep tests usually start in the evening. When you come to the sleep center, you are taken to a bedroom. You change into your nightclothes and lay on the bed. Next, a technician comes into your room and uses a special gel to paste about two dozen small, thin sensors on specific areas of your body: scalp, face, chest, and legs. Long, thin wires are attached to the sensors. The other ends of the wires go into a special machine called a polysomnograph in a nearby room. The sensors will measure your brain and muscle activity, eye movements, heart rate and rhythm, blood pressure, and how much air moves in and out of your lungs. An oximeter is often clipped on a finger or earlobe to measure the amount of oxygen in your blood during sleep. The polysomnograph will record the measurements.

The technician may turn on a video camera to record your movements and audio equipment to record snoring, talking, or other sounds you make during sleep. Finally, the technician turns on the sensors, turns off the lights, leaves the room, and you fall asleep. The sensors and wires do not usually bother people as they sleep. The sensors send data to a computer file as you sleep. When the test is finished in the morning, the technician removes the sensors, and you are able to go to school or go home.

Getting the Diagnosis

The sleep specialist will probably need a week or more to analyze your sleep test and other information. Then the doctor will talk with you about your results. You can talk by telephone or set up an appointment to speak in person.

The sleep specialist may tell you one of three outcomes. You may find out that you are sleeping more hours than you thought, and you don't have a sleep disorder. Or the sleep doctor may find explanations for your sleepiness, such as a disease or disorder, and may then refer you to a doctor specializing in your condition. If you are diagnosed with a sleep disorder, your sleep specialist will help you develop a treatment plan.

Getting Treatment

Sometimes, lifestyle changes are needed for people to sleep better and feel better. You will find information on lifestyle

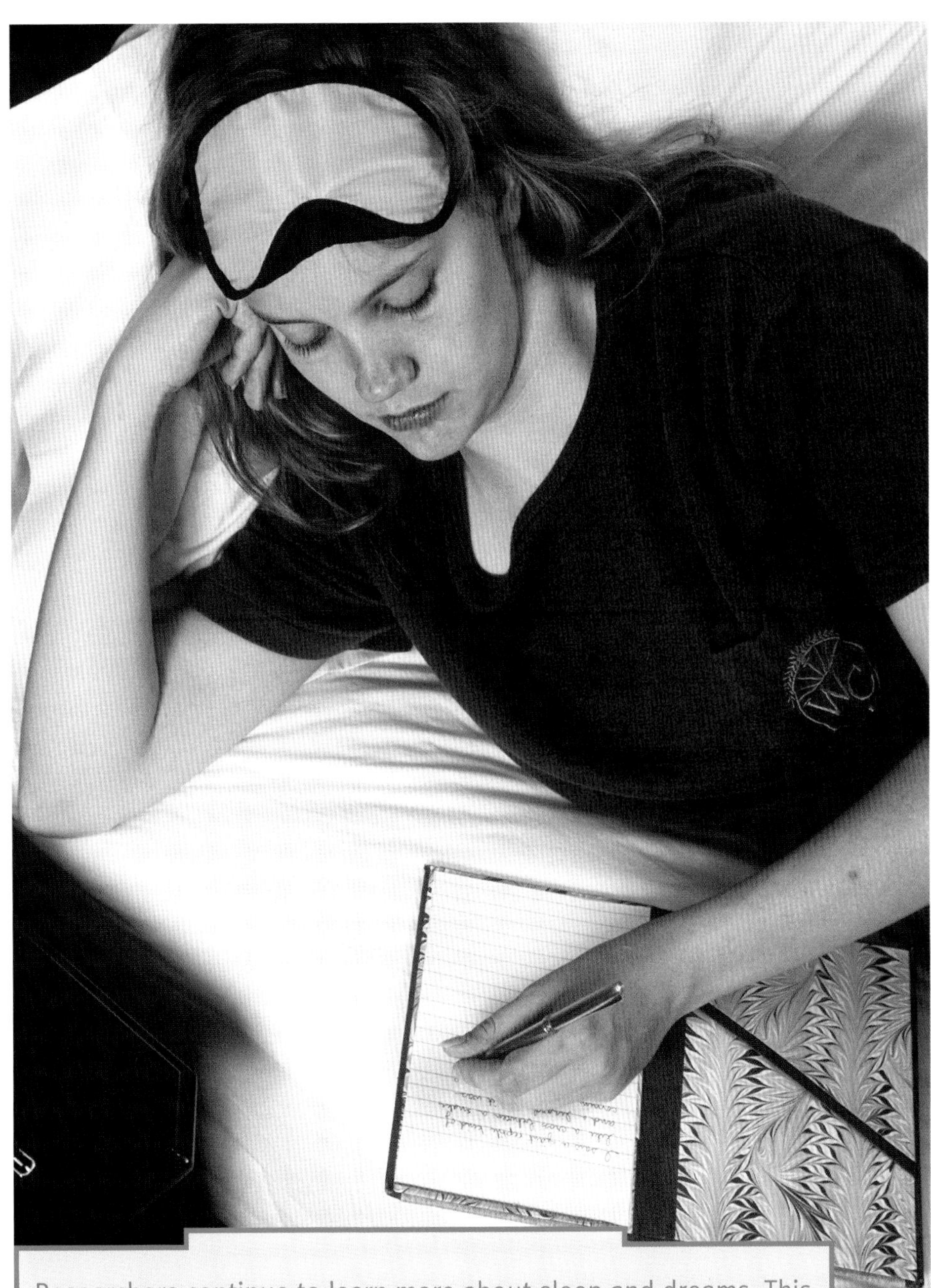

Researchers continue to learn more about sleep and dreams. This teen is part of a sleep experiment. She is recording her dreams in a notebook.

changes in the next chapter. Treatment like medication, devices, or therapy might be prescribed for your sleep problem or disorder. The following sleep problems or disorders typically require treatment.

Insomnia

People with chronic insomnia can often get help from a doctor or therapist. Most people who have insomnia can be helped with short-term medicine, or a combination of behavioral therapy and medicine. Sometimes, changes in sleep habits are all that is needed, such as not taking long naps during the day.

Doctors may prescribe an over-the-counter sleep aid or sleeping pills that are taken just before bed to treat insomnia for a short time. Most over-the-counter sleep aids contain an antihistamine that causes people to feel sleepy. However, people may feel sleepy during the day when they take antihistamines at night. Other side effects of antihistamines include dry mouth or feeling dizzy. Many newer prescription medications are designed to help people sleep and are not considered addictive. When monitored by a doctor, sleeping pills can be very effective. Sleep doctors may recommend cognitive behavioral therapy to help with insomnia. Cognition is the way in which you see your own reality and interpret your world. Cognitive therapy can help you change attitudes and beliefs that might be interfering with your sleep. Some people call this "sleep counseling."

People with chronic insomnia may require treatment for another problem, such as pain from arthritis or depression. Once pain from arthritis is controlled, people may sleep better.

Depression may need to be treated by a psychotherapist or psychiatrist.

Obstructive Sleep Apnea

Allergies, extra tissue in the throat or on the tongue, or enlarged tonsils can cause obstructive sleep apnea (OSA). Treating the allergy or removing the extra tissue or tonsils can cause the sleep apnea to disappear. Sometimes, OSA is due to obesity, so losing weight can reduce or eliminate the problem. For some people, doctors may prescribe a mouthpiece that adjusts the lower jaw

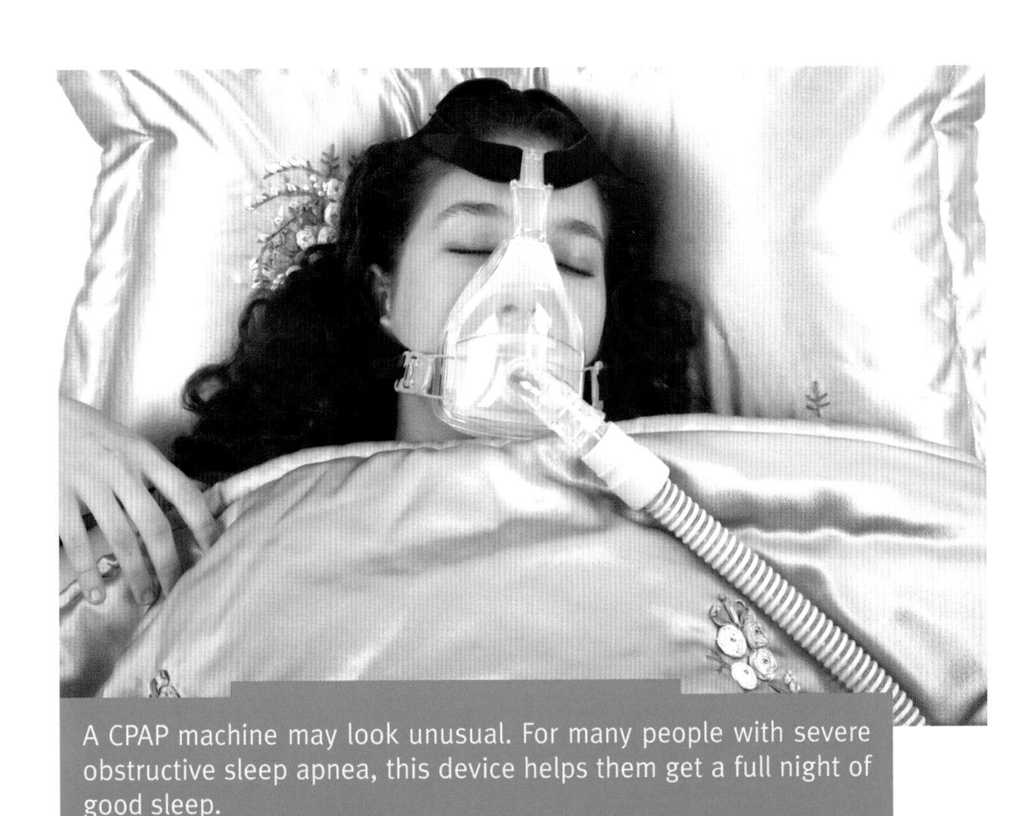

A CPAP machine may look unusual. For many people with severe obstructive sleep apnea, this device helps them get a full night of good sleep.

and tongue to keep the airway open. Using the mouthpiece helps prevent the collapsing of soft tissues in the throat that causes sleep apnea.

Doctors may prescribe continuous positive airway pressure (CPAP) for people with severe sleep apnea. CPAP is an air-pressure device connected by a hose to a mask that fits over the nose and mouth. The machine blows air through the mask into the airways. The flow of air forces the airways in your nose and mouth to stay open during sleep. The air pressure stays the same as you blow air in or out. By using this medical device, many people with apnea sleep well and wake up refreshed.

If you stop using CPAP, your sleep apnea will likely return. CPAP can irritate the nose or skin on the face and can cause headaches. Some people find the mask uncomfortable, or they dislike the cold air blowing on their face.

Sometimes, doctors will prescribe medications along with other treatments for sleep apnea. For example, certain antidepressants can help people with mild apnea.

Delayed Sleep Phase Syndrome

Counseling can help people learn to cope better with their delayed sleep phase syndrome. Therapists can help you learn to adjust your exposure to daylight, change the timing of your daily routines, and schedule short naps during the day. Bright light therapy might be helpful. This therapy adjusts your body clock by briefly exposing your eyes to safe levels of intense, bright light at scheduled times of the day. Your doctor may also prescribe sleeping pills to help you sleep at night or medications to help you stay awake during the day.

Restless Legs Syndrome

Researchers have found that RLS is more often seen in people who are deficient (lacking) some B vitamins and iron. To treat these deficiencies, doctors may prescribe iron or folate supplements or, rarely, vitamin B12 shots. If your RLS is painful, your doctor may prescribe pain relievers. He or she will determine if any of your medications, such as some allergy and cold medicines, are making your RLS worse. The U.S. Food and Drug Administration has not approved any drug to treat RLS, although researchers are studying some experimental drugs at this time.

Narcolepsy

Narcolepsy causes people to fall asleep too easily. Sleep doctors often prescribe medications to help, such as Modafinil, which decreases sleepiness during the day. Headaches are the most common side effects of this drug. If you have cataplexy (sudden loss of muscle power), your doctor may prescribe an antidepressant to decrease REM sleep.

Sometimes, people do not need medications or devices to deal with their sleep problems. They can get good sleep by making some changes in their everyday lives.

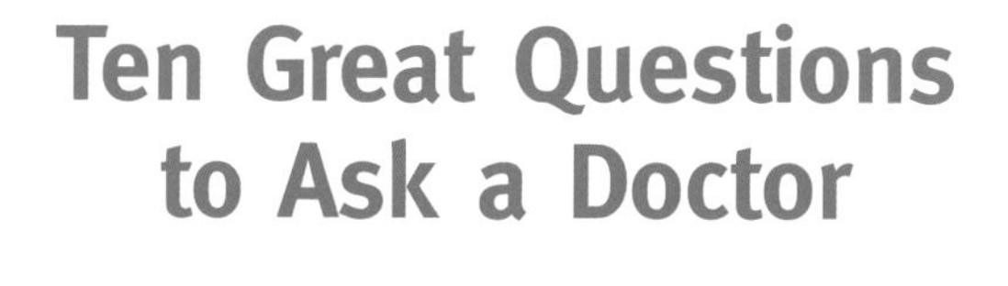

Ten Great Questions to Ask a Doctor

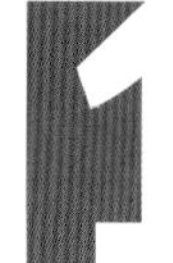

1. Do people yawn because they are not getting enough sleep?
2. Are sleep disorders inherited?
3. What colors in bedrooms help promote sleep?
4. Can drinking warm milk or eating baked turkey help me fall asleep?
5. Will loud music or opening the window keep me awake while driving?

6 Are sleep medicines addictive?

7 Can listening to self-help recordings during sleep help me learn?

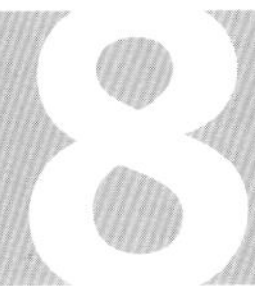

8 Can people quickly adjust to different sleep schedules?

9 Do people dream in color?

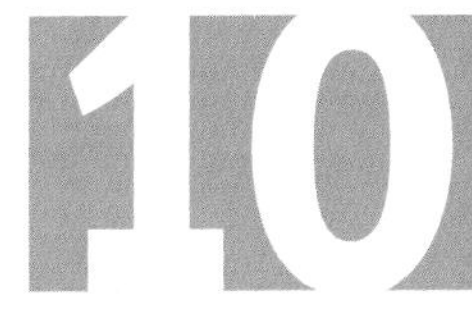

10 Is something wrong with me if I don't remember my dreams?

pt five

HOW CAN YOU GET A GOOD NIGHT'S SLEEP?

Getting enough sleep, eating a healthy diet, and exercising regularly are essential for good health. The best food or exercise program cannot make up for a sleep deficit or for poor sleep. Getting enough sleep is essential to your physical and mental health. Some factors that can affect sleep include when and how long you sleep, what you do before bedtime, and your sleeping conditions.

Make a Sleep Schedule

To help improve your sleep, make a regular sleep-wake schedule—and stick to it. Because teens usually require about nine hours of sleep every night, this leaves fifteen hours each day to do everything else. That may not sound like enough time for everything! However, one of the most important things you can do is plan your bedtime and sleep every day. Don't just go to bed whenever you happen to finish schoolwork, or e-mailing and text messaging your friends at night.

Every person has a different biological clock. Yours might be to stay awake until midnight. Because you live in the real world of school, schoolwork, and social activities, you may need to adjust your bed-wake times. For example, if your classes start at 7:00 AM and you need an hour to wake up, get ready for the day, and get to school, your wake-up time will be 6:00 AM. Going to sleep at midnight provides only six hours of sleep. To get a full nine hours of sleep, you should maintain a bedtime of 9:00 PM. You may find that you need to adjust your bedtime, but take a week or two to make the changes.

Try to stick to your sleep schedule, even on weekends. Your brain and body can probably handle an occasional night of not enough or poor-quality sleep. It's important to resume your usual sleep-wake schedule as soon as possible.

Before You Go to Bed

To help you fall asleep, plan your bedtime. If your prebedtime ritual is to wash up and leap into bed, you probably are not giving your brain and body enough time to transition to bedtime. As a result, you might still be thinking about an issue with a friend or parent as you try to fall asleep. Your body might be tense, and you cannot shut off thoughts about your problem.

To quiet your mind and relax your body, follow a calming bedtime routine. This helps you wind down from your busy day

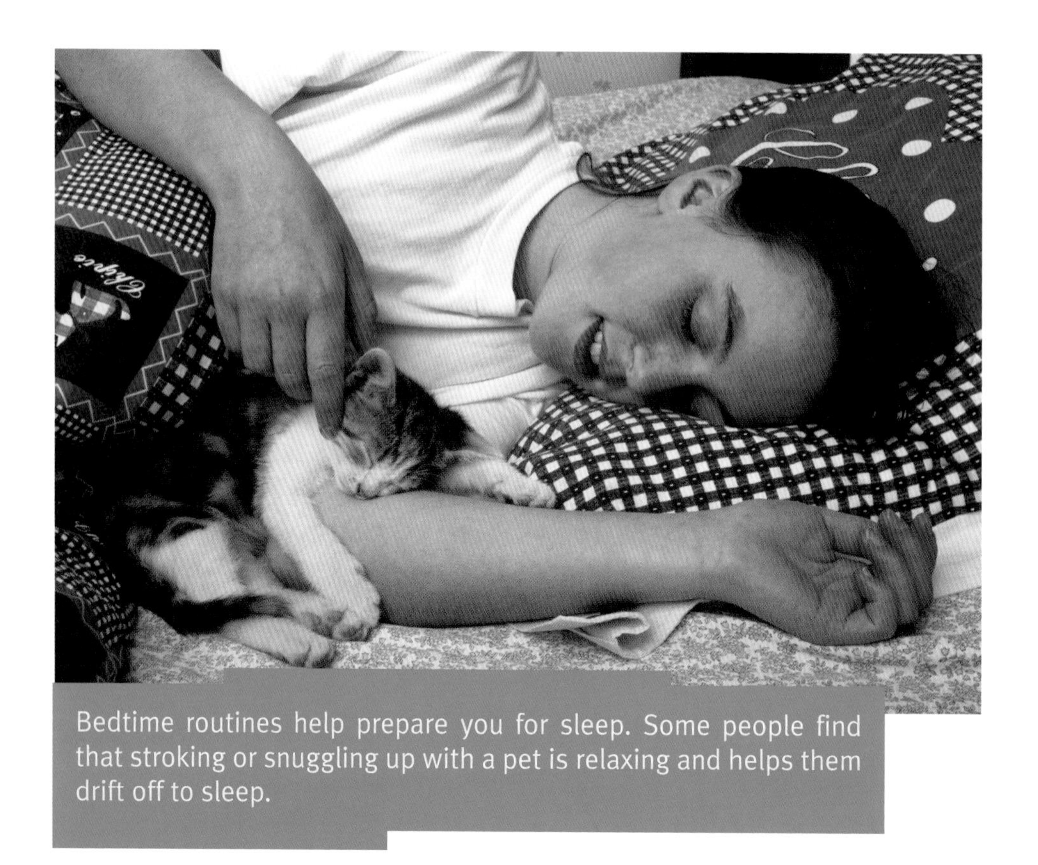

Bedtime routines help prepare you for sleep. Some people find that stroking or snuggling up with a pet is relaxing and helps them drift off to sleep.

and let go of stress and worries. Plan to take about thirty minutes to prepare for sleep. To start, turn off your computer, telephone, and television. Do something quietly that you will associate with bedtime. You might read an uplifting book, snuggle with a pet, play soft music, or take a warm shower or bath. Use your bed just for sleeping—not doing schoolwork, eating, or talking to your friends on the phone or text messaging.

Learn how to manage stress effectively. You can relieve stress by light stretching, deep breathing, or relaxation exercises. Some people like to imagine that gentle waves are rocking them to sleep, they are stretched out on a warm beach, or are laying under a large tree on a summer day. You can learn ways to manage stress through books, DVDs, or Web sites. Try different methods of stress management to find what works for you.

What to Limit or Avoid

You may have habits that are keeping you awake at night. For example, consuming too much caffeine in the afternoon or evening can cause difficulty falling asleep at night. Keep your daily limit of caffeine to the amount that is in two cups of regular coffee or two or three cans of caffeinated soda. Some energy drinks have more caffeine than four cups of regular coffee, so read labels or use the Internet to find information. Caffeine is also in teas, chocolate, coffee-flavored frozen desserts and gum, and some over-the-counter medicines. Some supplements contain herbs that are stimulants. If you are a heavy caffeine user, you might want to cut back. Do this gradually or you may feel irritable, tired, and have headaches.

If you often awaken to use the bathroom at night, limit your fluid intake during the evening. Some people eat a big meal or snack before bed. Your body digests food best when it's upright. When you are lying down, your body has more difficulty digesting food. This can lead to an upset stomach or reflux, which will disrupt your sleep. Reflux is the backing up of stomach acid into the throat and mouth.

To avoid reflux, eat two to three hours before bedtime and avoid fatty and spicy foods. You can also elevate the head of

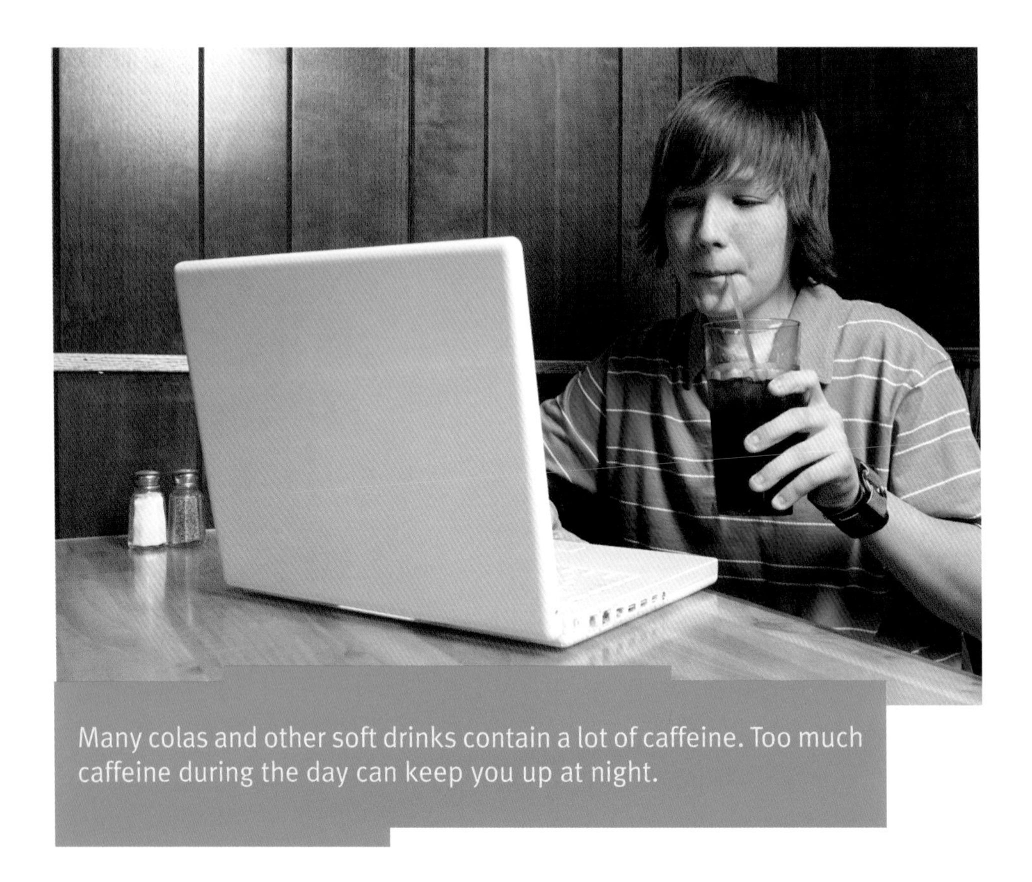

Many colas and other soft drinks contain a lot of caffeine. Too much caffeine during the day can keep you up at night.

your bed by putting bricks or sturdy blocks under the top legs of your bed to keep your head a little higher than your trunk during sleep. If you continue to have heartburn or reflux, see your family doctor.

Although you need regular exercise for good health, vigorous exercise close to bedtime increases your metabolism and brain activity. This may prevent you from relaxing to prepare for sleep. Try to exercise in the morning or five or six hours before bedtime. Exciting or disturbing video or computer games, television, surfing the Internet, or communications with friends close to bedtime can also keep you from falling asleep.

Some people think they sleep better with background noise, such as having the television on or music playing. Such noise actually disrupts sleep. White noise, though, can be helpful. You can run a white noise machine or a fan during the night. The sound of a whirling fan is similar to white noise and can help you sleep. You can also sleep with earplugs to block noise.

Changing Your Bedroom

You want your bedroom to be a restful and inviting place. To make the bedroom of your dreams, take some simple steps. First, clean your bedroom. You may not be able to fully relax if your room is dirty and your things are in piles everywhere. Tackle your piles by sorting through them and getting rid of items that you don't need or use anymore. Wash dirty clothes and put clean clothes away. Dust furniture, clean floors, and organize books, papers, DVDs, photographs, and other things.

Most people sleep best in cool temperatures. If your bedroom is too cool, wear socks to bed, put on a cap, or add another blanket. For a hot bedroom, lower the temperature or put on a fan.

Try not to fall asleep with a lamp or overhead light on. Light can disrupt your sleep cycles. Check that your window drapes, curtains, or shades block all outside light. If light remains, try to avoid having your bed face east so that the rising sun will not wake you. Cover the numbers on your electronic clock if they are too bright, or turn the clock around. You can also wear eyeshades to block out light.

Is your mattress lumpy or worn? You might need a new one. Many people find that a medium-firm mattress is most

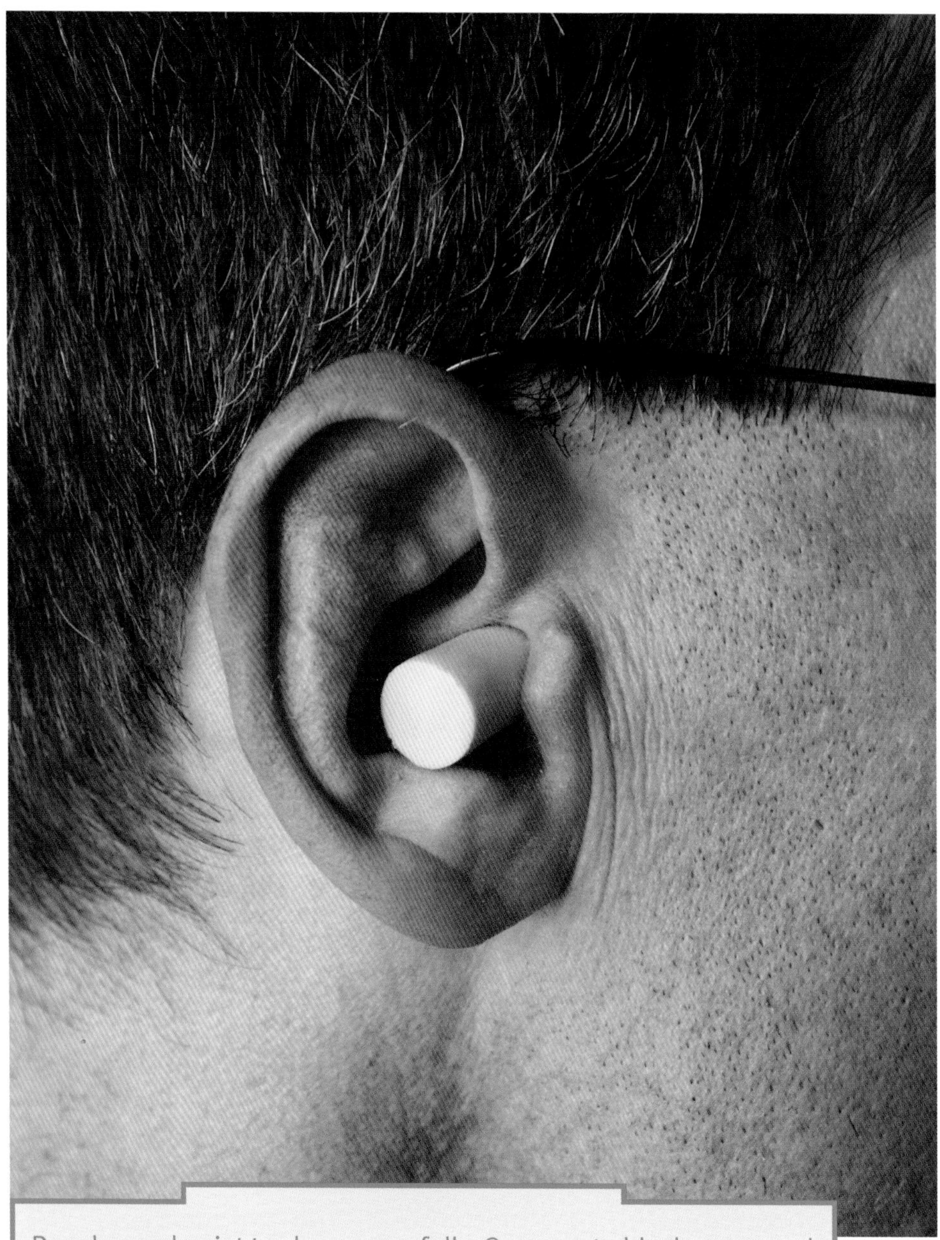

People need quiet to sleep peacefully. One way to block out sound is to use earplugs. They are available at many stores, often in the health and wellness aisle.

comfortable. Pillows wear out, too. If yours is flat or hard, find one that supports your head and neck and feels comfortable.

Sleep Tips

At bedtime, people tend to fall asleep within ten to twenty minutes. If you are still awake after twenty minutes, get out of bed and do a quiet activity in your room. Return to bed when you feel sleepy.

One way to deal with concerns is to write them down on paper, then put your list and a pen or pencil near your bed. Tell yourself that you don't need to think about your concerns during the night. This can stop your mind from dwelling on problems and help you fall asleep. If a new worry or idea comes up, jot down a quick note and go back to sleep.

Taking a nap during the day can be refreshing. Try to keep naps to twenty minutes or less because longer naps can affect nighttime sleep. Nap in the morning or early afternoon. A late-afternoon nap can cause you to be wide-awake at bedtime.

Regular exercise can help you sleep well because it relieves tension or stress. In addition, exercise often helps people fall asleep faster and sleep through the night. When you get enough sleep regularly, you may have fewer colds and find it easier to maintain a healthy weight. You won't feel as stressed, and you will be better able to cope with everyday events. Quality sleep will help you stay healthy and look and feel great.

Glossary

anemia A condition of low hemoglobin (the oxygen-carrying protein within red blood cells).

antidepressant A medication prescribed to treat depression and, sometimes, other health conditions.

biological clock A built-in system that keeps living things in time with the world around them.

cataplexy A sudden loss of muscle power ("collapse"), sometimes triggered by a strong emotion.

delayed sleep phase syndrome A sleep disorder in which the biological clock is delayed to a later sleep and wake-up time.

folate Folic acid, one of the B vitamins that is a main factor in the making of nucleic acid (DNA and RNA).

growth hormone A body chemical that stimulates the growth and repair of cells and tissues.

hallucination An imaginary sight, sound, or smell.

hormone A chemical in the body that affects the way other compounds or organs in the body behave.

insomnia The inability to fall or stay asleep, or the inability to sleep restfully.

melatonin A chemical produced by the pineal gland that is released when it's dark and helps make a person sleepy.

narcolepsy A serious sleep disorder characterized by very strong urges to sleep during the day. Someone with narcolepsy may also have paralysis upon awakening and hallucinations.

oximeter A physical sensor, usually attachable to a person's finger, which measures the amount of oxygen in the blood.

periodic limb movement disorder (PLMD) A condition characterized by brief, recurring jerks of the legs or arms.

pineal gland A small structure inside the brain that produces melatonin.

polysomnograph An instrument that records sleep patterns and bodily responses.

rapid eye movement (REM) sleep The portions of sleep during which a person dreams.

reflux The backing up of acid from the stomach into the throat and mouth.

restless legs syndrome (RLS) A condition characterized by a crawling, tingling, or creeping sensation in the legs that prompts a strong urge to move the legs to relieve the sensation.

sleep apnea A condition in which a person stops breathing periodically during sleep.

sleep cycle A series of stages, from light into deep sleep and then into REM sleep.

stimulant A drug that make people feel more awake and alert for a short time.

suprachiasmatic nucleus (SCN) The part of the brain that acts as a built-in body clock and helps control processes that go through a regular cycle of changes via secretion of melatonin.

For More Information

American Academy of Sleep Medicine
6301 Bandel Road, Suite 101
Rochester, MN 55901
(507) 287-6006
Web site: http://www.aasmnet.org
The American Academy of Sleep Medicine increases awareness of sleep disorders in public and professional communities.

American Sleep Apnea Association
1424 K Street NW, Suite 302
Washington, DC 20005
Web site: http://www.sleepapnea.org
(202) 293-3650
This association works to reduce problems stemming from sleep apnea and to help people with sleep apnea.

Better Sleep Council
501 Wythe Street
Alexandria, VA 22314-1917
(703) 683-8371
Web site: http://www.bettersleep.org
The Better Sleep Council educates about the importance of sleep to good health and quality of life.

Better Sleep Council Canada
P.O. Box 170
Streetsville, ON L5M 2B8
Canada
(416) 969-2809
Web site: http://www.bettersleep.ca
The council provides information about sleep.

Narcolepsy Network
10921 Reed Hartman Highway
Cincinnati, OH 45242
(513) 891-3522
Web site: http://www.narcolepsynetwork.org
This organization supports people with narcolepsy and increases public awareness of narcolepsy.

National Center on Sleep Disorders Research
National Heart, Lung, and Blood Institute
NHLBI Information Center
P.O. Box 30105
Bethesda, MD 20824
(301) 435-0199
Web site: http://www.nhlbi.nih.gov/about/ncsdr
The center promotes, maintains, and distributes information on sleep and sleep disorders.

National Highway Traffic Safety Administration
400 Seventh Street SW

Washington, DC 20590
(888) 327-4236
Web site: http://www.httsa.gov
This federal agency is charged with saving lives, preventing injuries, and reducing traffic-related accidents. Its Web site has information on teen drivers, including sleepy drivers.

National Sleep Foundation
1522 K Street NW, Suite 500
Washington, DC 20005
(202) 347-3471
Web site: http://www.sleepfoundation.org
The National Sleep Foundation works to improve understanding of sleep and sleep disorders, and by supporting sleep-related education, research, and advocacy.

Restless Legs Syndrome Foundation
1610 14th Street Northwest, Suite 300
Rochester, MN 55901
(507) 287-6465
Web site: http://www.rls.org
This foundation works to increase awareness, improve treatments, and through research, find a cure for RLS.

Sleep/Wake Disorders Canada
3080 Yonge Street, Suite 5055
Toronto, ON M4N 3N1

Canada
(416) 483-9654
Web site: http://www.pslgroup.com/dg/b538e.htm
Sleep/Wake Disorders Canada raises public awareness about sleep disorders and provides support for those with a sleep-wake disorder and their families.

Web Sites

Due to the changing nature of Internet links, Rosen Publishing has developed an online list of Web sites related to the subject of this book. This site is updated regularly. Please use this link to access this list:

http://www.rosenlinks.com/faq/sleep

For Further Reading

Bayer, Linda. *Sleep Disorders*. Philadelphia, PA: Chelsea House Publishers, 2001.

Covey, Sean. *The 7 Habits of Highly Effective Teens Personal Workbook*. Forest City, NC: Fireside Books, 2003.

Esherick, Joan. *Dead on Their Feet: Teen Sleep Deprivation and Its Consequences*. Philadelphia, PA: Mason Crest Publishers, 2005.

Esherick, Joan. *Drug Therapy and Sleep Disorders*. Philadelphia, PA: Mason Crest Publishers, 2007.

Espeland, Pamela. *Life Lists for Teens: Tips, Steps, Hints, and How-Tos for Growing Up, Getting Along, Learning, and Having Fun*. Minneapolis, MN: Free Spirit Publishing, 2003.

Fox, Annie. *Too Stressed to Think? A Teen Guide to Staying Sane When Life Makes You Crazy*. Minneapolis, MN: Free Spirit Publishing, 2005.

Hipp, Earl. *Fighting Invisible Tigers: A Stress Management Guide for Teens*. Minneapolis, MN: Free Spirit Publishing, 2008.

Hyde, Margaret, and Elizabeth H. Forsyth. *Stress 101: An Overview for Teens*. Breckenridge, CO: Twenty-First Century Books, 2007.

MacGregor, Rob. *Dream Power for Teens: What Your Dreams Say About Your Past, Present, and Future*. Cincinnati, OH: Adams Media Corporation, 2005.

Marcus, Mary Brophy. *Sleep Disorders.* New York, NY: Chelsea House Publishers, 2009.

Reber, Deborah. *Chill: Stress-Reducing Techniques for a More Balanced, Peaceful You.* New York, NY: Simon Pulse, 2008.

Rentz, Kristen. *YogaNap: Restorative Poses for Deep Relaxation.* Cambridge, MA: Da Capo Press, 2005.

Steinle, Jason. *Upload Experience: Quarterlife Solutions for Teens and Twentysomethings.* Evergreen, CO: Nasoj Publications, 2005.

Stewart, Gail B. *Sleep Disorders.* San Diego, CA: Lucent Books, 2003.

Index

About the Author

Judy Monroe Peterson has earned two master's degrees, including a master's in public health education, and is the author of more than fifty educational books for young people. She is a former health care, technical, and academic librarian and college faculty member; a biologist and research scientist; and a curriculum editor with more than twenty-five years of experience. She has taught courses at 3M, the University of Minnesota, and Lake Superior College. Currently, she is a writer and editor of K–12 and post–high school curriculum materials on a variety of subjects, including health, life skills, biology, life science, and the environment.

Photo Credits

Cover, pp. 23, 41, 52 Shutterstock.com; p. 5 © www.istockphoto.com/Zhang Bo; p. 9 © Hank Morgan/Photo Researchers, Inc; p. 11 © Volker Steger/Photo Researchers, Inc.; p. 14 © www.istockphoto.com/Bob Ingelhart; p. 17 © Picture Partners/Photo Researchers, Inc.; p. 19 © www.istockphoto.com/Thomas Eckstadt; p. 25 © www.istockphoto.com/Joshua Blake; p. 27 illustration © 2009 Nucleus Medical Art, all rights reserved, www.nucleus.com; p. 30 © Philippe Garo/Photo Researchers, Inc.; p. 35 pttmedical/Newscom; p. 39 © Will & Deni McIntyre/Photo Researchers, Inc.; p. 48 © Biosphoto/Klein J. L. & Hubert M. L./Peter Arnold Inc.; p. 50 © Image Source/Zuma Press.

Designer: Nicole Russo; Editor: Kathy Kuhtz Campbell;
Photo Researcher: Cindy Reiman

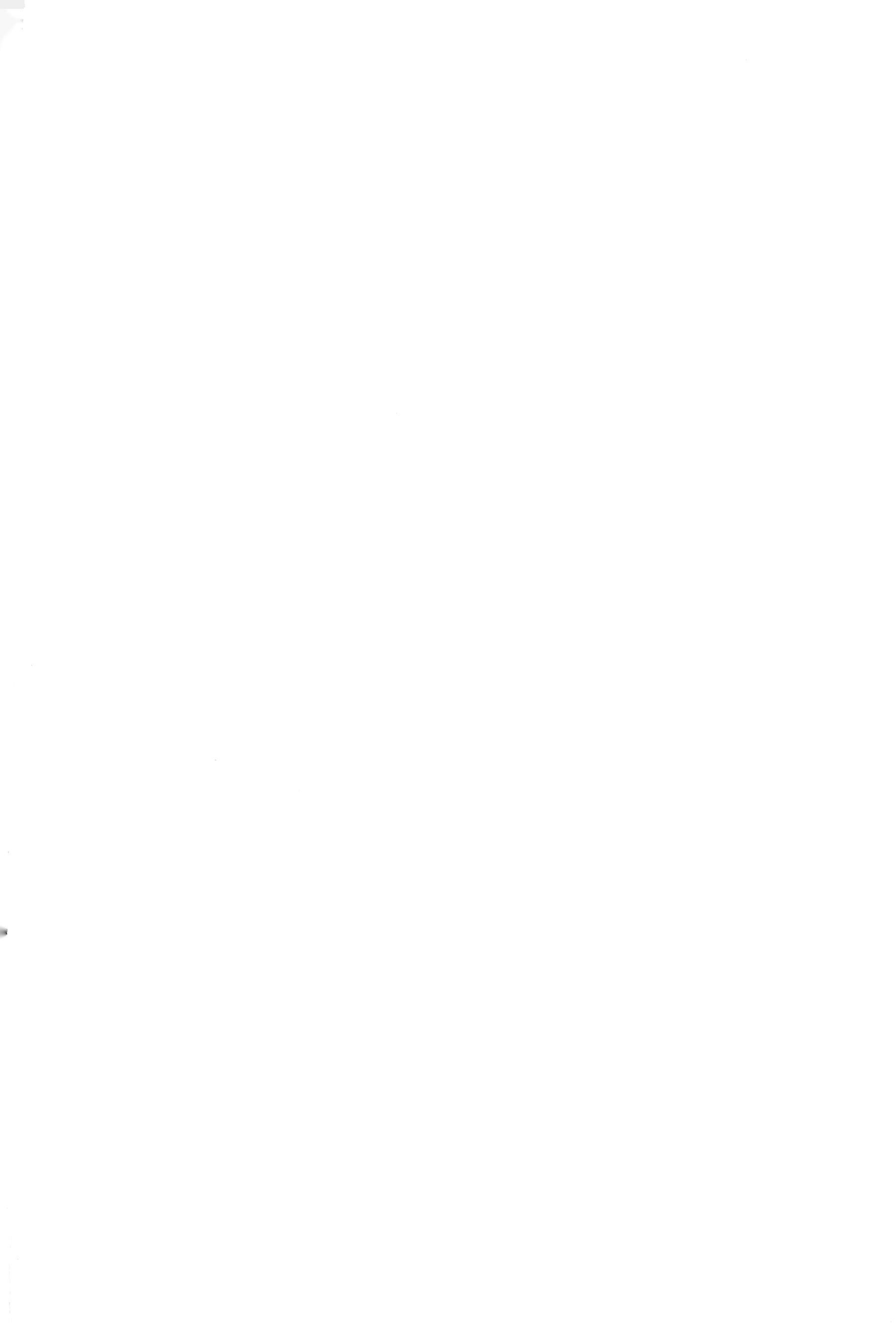